Narcissist

A Complete Step-by-Step Guide to Understanding and Healing from Emotional, Psychological Abuse and Unhealthy Relationships

Henna Rose

Contents

Introduction

I want to start off by commending you for finding this book. The fact that you picked it up shows that you are ready to take the beginning steps to recovery, which are some of the hardest steps to take. It's not easy to actively look for a way out and to look for a way to heal, particularly when one is under the dark and toxic cloud of abuse, but I believe that anyone who makes the effort to do so should be proud of themselves because it takes a great deal of strength to admit that something is wrong and it takes a great deal more to actually seek out a way to fix it.

Thank you for trying and striving for better because trust me when I say you deserve it.

There could be various reasons you are reading this book. It could be that you are in a relationship with someone who always needs attention and affection, but who ignores all your needs and feelings in turn. It could be that you know of someone who thinks they're holier than thou and you are tired of the constant expectation that they should be treated as if they're better than you and everyone else around you. It could be that you are tired of that one person who's always willing to serve insults in their condescending way, but heaven forbid you criticize anything they do because they're incapable of taking what they dish out. If any of these scenarios sound familiar, it's likely that you are dealing with a narcissist or two. Perhaps you are only now discovering what narcissists and gaslighting are. Maybe you know that you deal with narcissists every day and you are tired of it; you might have mere suspicions that you are looking to confirm or even deny, if that's the case. Whatever the case, I can help you through your journey into understanding what narcissists are, how they abuse us, and why they behave the way they do.

While narcissists are callous and cruel—and their behavior most often leads to lasting psychological trauma—the victim is not the only one suffering. Narcissism is a psychological disorder that exhibits itself in a manner of lashing out at others and inflicting lasting pain. It is a never-ending need for attention and reassurances, a fragile mask held up by little but a shaky scaffold. This does not excuse a narcissist's actions, as being a victim does not give you any reason to victimize another. A severe lack of sympathy, with little regard of empathy, together create the storm front that is the narcissist's personality and can easily swallow the unsuspecting into a world of lies, pain, and deceit.

It is likely that you find yourself turning these pages because you believe that you, or someone you know and care for, are suffering from within the confines of a narcissistic relationship. The fact that you have picked up this book is a good thing. This means you've reached your choice point—a moment in the cycle of narcissistic abuse in which a window is opened and you can use that window to escape or, at the very least, you are considering it.

While one has to maintain watch for a window to break free from a narcissistic relationship, falling into one is a concept much easier achieved. Narcissism is a giant pit-fall trap and, instead of politely waiting for you to step into it, the pit moves under you to consume you whole. Narcissists are a predatory lot; once they've set their ambitions on a goal, they stop at nothing to see that goal realized, uncaring of the wake of destruction they may leave in their path. The narcissist doesn't see the bond between two people in the same manner as a healthy individual does, instead they see what they can gain from that person or through knowing them, and they are willing to cast that person off at a moment's notice if it means achieving their goal.

If you are anything like me, that last one made you raise your eyebrows. Why on earth would you need to know why they behave that way? It's obviously unacceptable and that's all you need to know. On the contrary, a deeper level of understanding for the narcissistic personality disorder will help you in several ways. You will be able to spot them, you will be able to protect yourself from them, and you will be able to set up realistic and healthy boundaries for yourself.

Unlike becoming a victim of narcissism, which is terribly easy, breaking the cycle of damaging habits a friend, confidant, or partner has placed you in is a tougher journey. That's not to say the pathway you've found yourself on is impossible, at a crossroads torn between the comfort of familiarity and the peril of hope, but neither decision is easy to make. Either you choose the devil you know and return to the cold comfort of the manner in which a narcissist expresses their love, or you choose the devil you don't know and fight tooth and nail to return to a normal, happier life. After suffering from any kind of trauma, one can definitely find a long-term solution. The information in this book is here to help you heal, make your way toward a better place, and begin to live your life for yourself again. It's easy to lose ourselves to any kind of abuse and the most important part of recovering will be finding yourself again.

The struggle of fighting against an abuser can often feel like a lonely and tormented path—not only are you being isolated by the narcissist's behavior within that relationship, but it is easy to feel like you are doing this alone, that there is no one there for you, and that no one out there will understand. The truth is that you are not alone.

The sole purpose of this book is to show you that there is hope, a silver lining to the dark cloud that's been looming over your life, and that you are not alone. You are not the first, nor the last, to experience narcissistic abuse and as more cases are studied and breakthroughs are made in understanding this disorder, recognizing, handling, and healing from narcissistic abuse becomes easier to obtain and put into action.

If you are wondering how I'm so certain of all this, I'll tell you; I was just like you. I was abused for years not by one narcissist, but by several. You see, there's a direct link between narcissists and their victims. The most common type of relationship is generally one between a narcissist and someone who is codependent, but we'll get into that later in this book. The reason I share this is because narcissists have a type, which unfortunately means that people who fit within this personality type are often targeted and can have multiple experiences with narcissists throughout the course of their life rather than one— as if we needed more.

My point is that I know where you've been and if you take my hand, I'm going to lead and guide you out of that pit of despair and hopefully ensure that you never find yourself there again.

The material in this book is set out to instruct you on the characteristic hallmarks of narcissistic abuse and, by doing so, enabling you to recognize the signs of abuse. Recognition is the first step to acceptance, and acknowledgement is the first step toward healing. After you are able to uncover the pattern of narcissistic abuse, it is necessary to pinpoint and address the narcissist. The easiest way to stop the damage caused by a narcissist is to cut them out of your life, but that is not a possibility in every individual case. Sometimes the narcissist plaguing you is a colleague, someone within your family, or even that special someone you chose to spend the rest of your life with.

These points are a few topics that are elaborated on further within this book. By the end of this guide you will be able to confidently face down any trouble a self-absorbed narcissist cares to throw your way. On top of that, you will have the ability to overcome any damage sustained in dealing with a narcissist, most of the interaction simply washing by as you come to realize they're not as important as they think they are and that they are not worthy of your time. The more fragile relationships can be repaired—a bond between parent and child, two partners, or even just a close friend—instead of losing a connection to someone important to you.

While nobody is going to be able to take these steps for you, there will certainly be those in your corner rooting for you. You may be the one stuck in the struggle with an abusive partner, but your friends and family will push you to make the decision to put an end to your pain. Confide in those close to you and you will find someone willing to take each step of your recovery with you. It involves putting your trust into someone else, something that can be especially difficult for a victim of abuse, but it's a very necessary part of moving on. Support is a crucial aspect in your recovery process. Much like an addiction built over time, both the narcissist and the victim can begin to find a comfort and an attraction in the fragile dynamics built between them, and a friendly face or voice may be the only thing keeping you from sinking into that quicksand again.

A daunting task is set before you, one in which you hope to find a lasting peace in which you are allowed to heal and once again find yourself. You will learn about self-discovery, your identity, how to impress your desires onto the world by standing up for yourself. Along the way you will become equipped with the tools and knowledge that will protect you from falling into the victim role again and that will allow you to easily recover if you ever find yourself falling into that trap.

Most importantly, you will never have to endure suffering at the hands of another narcissist again. By the end of this book, you will have found freedom from narcissistic abuse and the toll it leaves on everyone involved. Let's begin taking those steps together.

Chapter 1.

Understanding Narcissism, Gaslighting, and the Role They Play in Your Life

One of the most important aspects, if not the most important aspect of healing from narcissistic abuse, is to understand the types of profiles narcissists actually exhibit (there are indeed various examples of narcissism and narcissists). The relevance comes in the fact that most narcissists suffer from a disorder, which is sometimes difficult to admit and accept. It can be easier to demonize the narcissists in your life, to simply regard them as being horrible people, rather than to delve deeper into the neuroscience behind their behavior. This would be a terrible and counterproductive thing to do. Without knowing the reason that narcissists act the way they do, it's easy to take all responsibility off of our own shoulders and the problem is that this weakens us. It makes us complacent in our positions in life when we are the only ones who can take the initiative to focus on healing ourselves instead of focusing on the wounds caused by the narcissists in our lives. Those actions begin with us. In order to avoid future narcissistic abuse, it's up to us to learn and recognize the symptoms and warning signs. All too often, the victims who have dealt with this personality disorder only find out that they are in an abusive relationship with equally abusive patterns when it is already too late because they simply weren't able to identify and catch the warning signs before the relationship reached that point.

You see, much like other personality and mental illnesses such as depression, anxiety, or bipolar disorder, the only way to know how exactly to proceed is to first learn. For example, when dealing with a person who has anxiety, there are certain actions and words that can trigger that person into feeling anxious. If you had a better understanding of the way anxiety worked, however, you would find yourself able to avoid causing and exacerbating the person's anxious tendencies. Beyond that, you would be able to not only assist them in treating their disorder, but assist yourself in coping with it too.

The fact of the matter is those with mental illnesses and personality disorders are not the only ones who suffer from their ailment—though to them, it can feel that way. They don't always realize the impact that they have on the people around them, both dear to them and not. It's due to this lack of self-awareness, and the fact that people suffering from mental illnesses are generally treated with a larger sense of severity, that the negative effects exhibited on or by the people around them are often ignored, not properly addressed, and hardly ever considered to be in need of resolving. While treating those with mental disorders is important, it's just as important to ensure that the people around them—be it family members, employers/employees, friends, or partners—are receiving proper treatment too. They should be given an explanation of the disorder, coping and recovery methods for themselves, and a few lessons in the correct approach for particular patterns of behaviors.

Unfortunately, getting outsiders to see and agree that this is the best way forward is far easier said than done. You don't have to worry about that though. That's why I'm here; to better explain what exactly narcissists are, why they are the way they are, and how you can move toward a better place as a result. These identification guidelines will help you cope with current narcissistic presences in your life, recover from past experiences with narcissistic abuse, and spot the signals before you find yourself caught in that vicious cycle again.

So, What Is a Narcissist?

Before any healing can take place, it is necessary to come to an understanding of what you are dealing with and exactly what you are going through. By definition, narcissism is a mental disorder. It's commonly referred to among practitioners as being 'pathological self-absorption' and while it has existed since Ancient Greece, it was only identified as a mental disorder in 1898 by Havelock Ellis, a British essayist and physician. Narcissism has a long history, having been touched on even by Sigmund Freud at one stage. The term 'narcissist' has also been used to describe having feelings about oneself that one might ordinarily have had for a sexual partner. That in itself speaks volumes about the level of self-absorption that narcissists can harbor. Narcissistic personality disorder (NPD) is a complex mental disorder forming part of a cluster of disorders; these are characterized as having wildly emotional thinking or behavior which often leads to unpredictable actions and consequences.

Unlike most mental disorders, narcissists may not feel that they are suffering, but their personality disorder can cause issues in various areas of their life. For one thing, they can feel unhappy purely because they aren't getting the attention they feel they deserve. Put simply, narcissists have massive egos. Their sense of self-importance is inflated and their compulsive self-absorption plays a major part in how and why their other tendencies exist. I'm sure you've heard the term, "They need to boost their ego." Well, if that expression wasn't first said about a narcissist, it should have been.

My experience has been that narcissists feel the need to feed their ego. More than that, they want someone else to tell them that they're amazing. This can come in the form of words or in joining their condescending laughter even if you don't necessarily find their behavior funny. For the most part, the narcissist requires validation and has an excessive need for attention and/or admiration. They lack any sort of empathy for people around them and this causes them to have condescending and superior attitudes. When I didn't laugh, my abuser went into an episode of silence that spoke louder than anything they could have said to me. I could feel the disappointment emanating off of them. The worst part was that I knew this wouldn't fade away; if it wasn't made up for in some way, it would eventually blow up later on.

Now, there's a lot more to narcissism than ego, but that's one of the biggest points of their personalities, usually accompanied by a superiority complex. Contrary to the belief that they have an extreme sense of self-confidence, narcissists actually have very fragile self-esteem. It's all an act, a set of armor that they wear to coerce and manipulate their way into being treated the way they want to be treated. This is one of the root causes of their behavior. When they aren't validated the way that they want to be, they grow disappointed and unhappy, usually becoming so negative that no one actually wants to be around them. Their fragile self-esteem means that they are vulnerable and the slightest hint of criticism can lead to adverse reactions. In essence, they're a bomb waiting to explode.

Unfortunately, this puts people like you and I right in the line of fire. Narcissists will not see this deep-seated need and the resounding response as something that they themselves can stop, nor will they see that they are the cause of their own unhappiness. Rather, they will blame those around them for not feeding into the admiration and attention that they so crave. They may find their relationships unfulfilling, which can lead to a myriad of other atrocities committed such as unfaithfulness, lies, and emotional or other forms of abuse.

What Is Gaslighting?

At some point in our lives, each of us figures out who we are at our core. Then, out of nowhere, we begin doubting ourselves, questioning motives, and second-guessing things. Quickly, our confidence can transform into paranoia and suspicion. A lack of self-esteem can cause us to become high-strung.

When this happens, it's hard not to blame ourselves and think that we're losing our minds, but if you recognize any of these feelings that you never used to be as familiar with, you might be a victim of gaslighting. In order to gain control and power over a person and a relationship, a person will begin to use manipulation to plant seeds of doubt into their victims. This happens over time and can be hard to immediately spot, but eventually the victim will be so consumed with self-doubt that they begin to question their own reality.

Does this sound familiar? That's because narcissists and other abusers use gaslighting and as we know, it's not always easy to spot these individuals. To make matters worse, gaslighting is used in a slow manner, deliberately ensuring that the victim doesn't realize what is happening to them. Narcissists and gaslighting have many things in common, one of which being that they're both so charming that it's hard to recognize the abuse and the lies. In fact, guilt might be one of the emotions you feel when you second-guess this character. Confusion is the gaslighter's aim and so, they use certain tactics to prove you wrong to the point where you start to ignore your gut.

In 1944, a film called *Gaslight* was released. It's the perfect way to define gaslighting and is the source of its name. The plot is that a husband brainwashes his wife until she thinks she's going clinically insane. While fighting to protect the identity that her husband tried to take, the wife was still exhibiting some symptoms of Stockholm Syndrome. Due to the amount of uncertainty instilled into victims by their abusers, they become dependent on their gaslighter.

The signs of gaslighters include:

- Confusion, as mentioned above, is one of the tools gaslighters use. They rely on the fact that people crave stability. Most often, victims turn to their abusers for clarity in the face of confusion, thereby increasing the power of the abuser, the very person ensuring that they are constantly confused.

- Gaslighters tell lies so obvious that you know it, but they do it with such ease that you begin questioning the simplest things and that's where the self-doubt starts.

- They deny things and even though, once again, you know what they said/did, they deny it and ask you to prove it when you only have your own memory to go on. With enough force, you can begin to second-guess yourself. You'll start accepting their reality and questioning yours.

- Hooking their claws even further into you, you may find that the gaslighter takes issue with the things you hold dear to the point that the foundations on which you built yourself are things you begin to question—from your favorite color to your dream job to whether you should have had children.

- Words mean nothing when it comes to gaslighters. They like to talk, but their actions reveal more about the underlying issues. How do they treat the victim?

- Narcissists aren't the only ones who like to build you up and then break you down. It's a trick to keep you holding on. Their praise and approval leads you to believe that they aren't as bad as you think they are when you are being torn down, made worse by the fact that you grow used to it.

- You may find that you defend yourself for things you didn't do in this type of dynamic because the gaslighter projects their own actions onto you, accusing you of things like lying and cheating because it's what they're doing.

- By now, you can start to see how the manipulation takes time to turn the victim into someone else. The most confident humans can turn into mere shells of what they once were, while remaining totally unaware of what is happening. Their reality diminishes entirely.

- While you question your sanity, they'll hammer the nail in your coffin by calling you crazy and telling others you are crazy. Since you are already searching for clarity in them, you believe their words. Worse still, if you ever tried to get help, other people wouldn't believe you because the gaslighter has already told them it would happen and that your craziness means you shouldn't be taken seriously.

- This makes it easy for your abuser to convince you that everyone is against you. You may start to believe everyone you come across is a liar, further blurring your sense of reality. It causes you to turn to them once again, thereby allowing the cycle to continue.

Now that you know these signs, it will be easier for you to spot them. The next time you find yourself questioning whether or not the person standing in front of you should be trusted, go with your gut before it's too late. There's a reason humans have instincts and out of all the animals on earth, we're the only ones who not only second-guess them but who third and fourth-guess them too.

Remember that not every person you fight with or question is going to be a gaslighter or narcissist, but be sure to keep track and the second you start to feel like something is wrong, take action. You can turn to someone you trust for a second opinion if necessary. The quicker you spot these techniques, the better your chances of maintaining your own reality and avoiding the pattern of abuse.

The reason you need to keep track is because the abuser turns your reality around and once you start losing that perception, you become confused. You have to confirm that what's happening is actually gaslighting in order to move forward. Use the steps to self-care found in this book to help you stay grounded if your reality comes into question.

The Neuroscience Behind Narcissism

The reason it is necessary for an individual to educate themselves about narcissism and how to distinguish that particular behavior from others is due to its complexity in nature, as well as similarities between the symptoms presented in these other disorders. The capacity of the human brain is immense and we've barely scratched the surface of how it all works together, in spite of the advancements made in research—and that's only speaking about it in its healthy state. Once damage and trauma is thrown on top of an already complicated system, it becomes a nightmare to diagnose, let alone fix, but the good news is that people are trying.

As new cases are brought forward and medical professionals are able to study its facts, new parallels can be drawn. Patterns start to form and a cohesive picture of the problem reveals itself to you. The extent of narcissistic personality disorder is vast and we only have fragments of the whole image. We don't have every answer about NPD, and we probably won't for some time, but there is currently enough understanding to help you break the bonds of narcissism and heal from your wounds.

Narcissism stands out from the other disorders in its cluster—those being antisocial personality disorder, borderline personality disorder, and histrionic personality disorder—by their entitlement and expectations. While these disorders can share signs such as irrational rage, wild emotions, acts of violence, or abnormal social behavior, the reasons each disorder causes those specific outcomes is different.

Due to the similarities, each disorder has received its own criteria to establish whether or not someone is suffering from that specific ailment, or one of the many disorders like NPD. For each set of criteria, an individual must exhibit a certain amount of those signs to be diagnosable with that type of disorder. NPD has nine criteria, but we will expand on that further down.

Peeling back the layers behind what makes the narcissist tick, alongside learning their cues, will allow you to create a semblance of rationality behind the actions the narcissist takes and stymie some of the energy behind their attacks. If you don't give them what they're looking for, you take the wind right out of their sails. It has often been the best course to first understand your adversary before taking action, simply because the understanding will make clearer paths of legitimate options. Instead of flailing in the dark, this understanding will be a light to guide your way.

There is a difference between being a narcissist and suffering from narcissistic personality disorder. It sounds strange, but there are simply egoistic beings out there that, whilst exhibiting some of the traits of narcissism, cannot be identified as sufferers of a personality disorder. To use the example from before, a person can be anxious even if they do not suffer from an anxiety disorder. That's why evaluations are performed when narcissists are treated for their personality disorder—to be certain that that's what it is, as well as to find out what treatment plan is applicable and suitable.

The narcissistic personality disorder is sometimes characterized by surface-level behavior. They'll carry that same arrogance and confidence we're familiar with, but beneath that, they are sensitive and filled with shame and guilt. These people don't function well in society and generally alienate themselves from friends and family, which can lead to depression and isolation. People with the disorder are caught between their feelings of superiority and their feelings of gloom all at once.

The unfortunate thing here is that their mental disorder makes it difficult to admit that anything is wrong with them.

Meanwhile, the narcissist often has no such qualms. They have superior and arrogant attitudes, but they see nothing wrong with treating people as if they are less. In fact, they're so obnoxious that their lack of empathy makes them immune to concern for the plights of others. The only feelings they care about are their own. This is why it's easy for them to exploit other people to get what they want and as entitled as they are, they'll look down on people who show them appreciation. They lack self-awareness and for that reason, they show no remorse, unlike the sufferers of the personality disorder, who are filled with shame. Lying, for one thing, is something that comes easily and almost compulsive to the narcissist.

Narcissists chase power, money, and prestige. They will do anything to obtain it, even if that means using or hurting people along the way. Too many of them succeed, including a vast amount of past and present world leaders such as Adolf Hitler. On the other hand, their counterparts who suffer from a legitimate mental disorder hide from the world and boast their mask of confidence in public.

Neuroscientific Observations of Narcissism

The truth is that there isn't a lot of information on this disorder as of yet. There are several common factors that come up in the various tests that *have* been performed thus far, but self-diagnostic tools and psychological evaluations have been the way forward as it has only recently begun to be taken seriously as a disorder. For the moment, talk-therapy is the most recommended treatment plan available to sufferers and is probably one of many steps that those recovering from the abuse of a narcissist would first take, but there have been several tests and brain scans done in an effort to understand narcissism.

- Of the few existing studies on narcissistic personality disorder, one of the consistent notions is that narcissism points to irregularity in certain areas of the brain, especially in the insular cortex (Journal of Psychiatric Research, 2019). This is one of the parts of the brain responsible for cognitive control, also known as the ability to override impulses and make conscious decisions. What we can deduce here is that this is where the beginnings of a lack of empathy and a tendency toward sadism comes from.

- Until further tests and studies are conducted, we won't know the exact cause, but it's presumed that environmental factors play a role. These could include biological, psychological, and social factors. The nature versus nurture argument comes to mind, but that has never fully been resolved to a definite answer and the same can be said for narcissism. There's a chance that narcissists are simply born with different brain chemicals from the rest of us as much as there is a chance that the way they were raised is the reason they are the way they are.

- It's highly likely that every human is capable of being a narcissist. The key factor in determining healthy from pathological is the extent to which a person is narcissistic. An assessment is usually completed using interviews, self-reports, or even projective tests where one reacts to ambiguous stimuli in the hopes that they reveal some form of hidden emotions or conflicts. The truth is that we all have selfish and arrogant predispositions, but what discerns pathological from healthy is the ends to which we hold those leanings.

- Part of the narcissist's brain patterns is that they tend to have multiple features of their disorder. That is to say, it's rare, if not downright impossible, that you will ever come across a narcissist who exhibits a single one of the core dimensions. At first, it was believed that there was only one way of defining a narcissist, which is to say that they're self-absorbed. Further conducted studies revealed instead that it is a multidimensional disorder, inclusive of grandiosity and attention-seeking.

- In a way, narcissism resembles other known psychiatric disorders such as autism and borderline personality disorder. How, you ask? It all lies in the brain activity. The insular cortex is associated with disgust, emotional processing, intuition, awareness, uncertainty, and overstepping boundaries—if you've ever experienced a narcissist for yourself, this will resonate with you since these are common emotions that it seems narcissists are either unfamiliar with or which cause them to behave abnormally compared to other people. It also relays certain feelings such as pain, touch, and itches, thereby allowing for the awareness of feelings. Persons with unusual activity in this area of the brain can have strange patterns or reactions outside of the norm—as seen in the autistic spectrum and, as I'm sure you've noticed, in narcissists.

- So, too, the brain is affected in terms of empathy. It has been observed in those with narcissistic personality disorder that the thickness of their cerebral cortex was lesser than standard. It's believed that the reduction of gray matter in this area is directly related to empathy and this can explain why it's so easy for narcissists to exploit and manipulate other people without feeling remorse.

- Narcissists are believed to be high-functioning, most commonly because they're ambitious. This is why it's not always seen as impairment, especially in the narcissist's own eyes. On the contrary, many successful people are narcissistic, so why would they believe it's a bad thing? That being said, while confidence can lead to success, it's important to note that the arrogance of a narcissist can make them unwilling to compete with others while their low self-esteem could hold them back from taking risks due to the fear of failure. Their lack of empathy can prove them difficult to get along with in various areas of life, especially professional environments where teamwork is almost always a key factor in succeeding.

- These individuals are often disarmingly charming, which is one of the forms of manipulation and coercion that they use, and this is why it's difficult to notice the abnormalities at first. They're the type of people who draw you in and their cool exterior, overwhelming confidence, and ability to say the exact right thing at the right time all play into the trap. We can take away from their unusual insular cortex that, in conjunction with their lack of empathy, they have trouble with higher processing such as making decisions and judgments.

The Physiology and Cause of Narcissism

Several aspects have been linked to the development of narcissism, including nurture received during upbringing, genetic predispositions to the disorder, and a variety of obstructions in the working of the brain and neural pathways. It is common for narcissists to exhibit a smaller left anterior insula cortex in the brain—MRI scans showing less gray matter in that structure within people suffering from narcissistic personality disorder—and researchers have linked this area of the brain as crucial to feeling empathy.

However, the researchers clearly state that this area of the brain is not the only part responsible for the feeling of empathy (Journal of Psychiatric Research, 2019). As many areas of the brain play a few key roles, they also handle a myriad of secondary and tertiary tasks and so narcissists are still capable of recognizing what other people are feeling or thinking—despite this, they show little to no concern as to how those emotions and desires impact that individual, but rather they see the individual as a complex puzzle or pattern and once the narcissist sees what it is, they can maneuver through it to get to their own needs.

As much as narcissism stems from a lack of empathy, which can be linked to an underdeveloped neocortex, much of the behavior and cues a narcissist exhibits are deeply rooted in other areas of the brain. The brain consists of two distinct areas separated primarily based on the functions they provide and the roles they serve within one's own body and conscious, as well as the individual's role in society.

Along with key roles in the sensory input and output of our bodies, the primal or reptilian brain, comprised of both the basal ganglia (or brain stem) and the limbic system, serves to provide the survival instincts necessary for the survival of ourselves, those close to us, and our species. These often pertain to providing food, reproduction, as well as being the seat for the decision on whether to fight or flee. Communication from the primal brain is often expressed physically as opposed to languages.

The neocortex is centered around higher thought, pertaining to reasoning and logic as well as the understanding and communication through language. Insight and empathy are closely tied to the processes that take in this higher functioning part of the brain.

Narcissists have been shown to suffer a structural abnormality in their neocortex and often fall back on the structures within the primal brain. Their social interactions can often be wolfish and undermining, and that ties into exactly where their intention and action is coming from. The fight or flight system is found within the amygdala, part of the limbic system, and controls whether or not to engage in a situation and stand your ground but risk losing something, or to be done with the situation as soon as possible and flee—often sacrificing something meaningful to do so.

Narcissists prey on this instinct in others, often inciting shame or fear to trigger a reaction. Any reaction on that level will normally play into a narcissist's hands—they're experienced at this, and once you are flustered you won't be able to pull together a proper mental defense without taking a moment to collect yourself.

One of the side effects of narcissistic abuse is an enlarged amygdala. Handling the fight or flight reactions in our bodies, an enlarged amygdala will cause the brain to rely more heavily on its function, bringing that response to the fore more often than a logical response. This begins to affect actions in everyday life, even if the narcissist isn't present. A bowl dropping to the floor triggers the response before your brain can tell you it was just a bowl, and you are on edge—a colleague popping their head around your office door to give you a reminder, as they usually do, and that sets your heart racing.

There are ways to recover from this mindset, generally through similar counseling as post-traumatic stress disorder (PTSD) sufferers. Continued exposure to narcissistic abuse can cause the victim to develop PTSD or C-PTSD—complex post-traumatic stress disorder. To better handle these topics and how to recover from the abuse, more information will be provided later in a chapter dedicated to healing.

Call to Action

When it comes to narcissism and narcissistic abuse, it is up to you to make the decision to move on and heal from the pain. The narcissist is getting what they want, so they will happily keep chugging along with their usual to-do. There will come a time in the cycle of abuse where you have a gap to get out—it's called the choice-point—and the only way you can utilize that moment is by knowing that you are dealing with a narcissist and understanding the behavior they're putting you through.

Many people suffer through abuse at the hands of a narcissist, completely oblivious to what they're experiencing. There are some who'll understand that abuse is going on and that the person is toxic for them, but they won't understand why. Heck, even people who know about narcissism might not realize they're dealing with a narcissist, or how exactly they should deal with the narcissist in turn.

If you feel like there is something off in a relationship that is constantly a burden, making you feel drained, has left you hurt and ashamed, or is making you doubt yourself, you should take a closer look at that relationship. Instead of being caught unaware when the narcissist comes looking for something, you will know exactly who you are dealing with.

Set some time aside to reflect on the people that are close to you and mean something to you. Compare their personalities and actions to the traits and behavior of a narcissist. Keep in mind, a person must exhibit the traits over a period of time and they must exhibit five or more traits to potentially be suffering from NPD.

For those who meet many of the narcissistic conditions, we will handle in-depth processes on how to approach or deal with these narcissists. For the most part, recognizing the pattern of behavior and denying the narcissist at the choice-point allows you to exit the abuse cycle. The narcissist will attempt to reestablish the same cycle so you will have to remain on your guard. Don't let them snake their way back into a damaging position in your life.

If the narcissist in question plays only a small role in your life, you can cut them off, or at least minimize your contact with them. You have options you can take, a way to permanently cut the narcissist off. You may not even have to deny them on the regular. Those in familial or intimate relationships with you may take a lot more care and a completely different approach, especially if you want to maintain the connection with a parent, a child, or a spouse.

If, instead, the individual exhibits only a few signs of narcissism and the behavior that goes alongside this, you can assert yourself and address the issues you have with them. The behavior is still toxic, but if you can reach an understanding about what their behavior does and how it makes you feel, that individual is likely to change their behavior. Don't approach them as an accuser, but rather as someone damaged.

I also stress that this option is not always a wise course with someone suffering from full blown narcissistic personality disorder as their fragile mindset can turn them aggressive under a confrontation, as civil as it may be. If the narcissist feels undermined, they will become defensive and lash out if pushed.

The Traits of Narcissists

Narcissists are nothing if not eye-catching. Think of a human peacock and you will begin to get the image of a narcissist—though there are some peacock humans out there who don't qualify as narcissists, no matter how arrogant or flamboyant they may be. Alongside this alluring show of bright and colorful feathers and an over-indulgent sense of self-confidence, narcissists have an empathetic void which prevents them from concerning themselves with the needs or desires of others.

While we know a fair amount about narcissism, there is a vast amount that is left as of yet unknown to us. The cause of narcissism hasn't been agreed upon by experts—that is to say there isn't any certain proof that can be accepted to fulfill the cause of narcissism—but it can appear as early as the teenage years. That being said, any individual is likely to have encountered one or more narcissists by the time they've reached their late twenties, and you may not have been aware of what was happening at the time. Despite not understanding, the experience would still leave you wrecked, damaged, and unsure of yourself. The thing about psychological and emotional abuse is that they're some of the hardest to pinpoint without that understanding. It can go unchecked for a while before you realize what's happening and the damage that it's inflicting, which is why it often happens that the victim is abused for a long time before reporting or attempting to do something about it. The key is learning what the characteristics are so that the timeframe for which you tolerate them is shortened.

These characteristics have to be prevalent across a variety of traits for an individual to be considered narcissistic, and excessively so for someone to be diagnosed with NPD. Narcissistic personality disorder and narcissism differ slightly, but only in the extent of each characteristic related to the personality traits. Behind these walls of ego and altruism lies a very fragile core to the narcissist, and any danger posed to this fragile self-image hidden behind their grandiosity will cause a narcissist to become prickly. Rejection, disinterest, and other actions many narcissists evoke are considered attacks when they are faced with the same arsenal they use. A narcissist appears to be collected and composed on the surface, but beneath lies a broiling pool of hate, self-loathing, anger, and a myriad of other emotions, most of which are equally negative.

Take a moment to consider that. Remember when I said that it's important to accept that the narcissist is also suffering? We have to remember that in spite of their behavior, this person is still another human being. That's not to excuse their words or actions, but it does allow us, beings perfectly capable of feeling the empathy they lack, to imagine what it would be like in their shoes. In order to move on, one has to be able to forgive. Perhaps forgiveness will come to you in the knowledge that such negativity is all-consuming. Can you imagine being filled with that much loathing? I don't know about you, but that sounds exhausting and sad to me. Narcissists need treatment as much as their victims do.

Like any personality disorder, narcissism requires certain criteria to be met before a personality aligns with the disorder. There are two models that, while bearing similarity in the respective areas each considers, proposed two alternative methods to determining the structure of a narcissistic personality.

The first method is the most commonly cited idea, proposing that of nine criteria, at least five should be present within an adolescent or adult to establish a case for narcissistic personality disorder:

- Primarily this idea focuses around an over-inflated self-importance. Their well-being and opinion are not only their primary concern, but it should be put above those of others.

- Narcissists are dreamers and they are often caught in the midst of aggrandizing themselves in their latest fantasy. They preoccupy themselves with visions in which they are surrounded by lavish richness, or they have immense power that they can exert to see their whim come to life, or bathing in the admiration and recognition of others, or they are lost in the arms of their latest true love—destined not to last.

- The narcissist believes that he or she forms part of an elite crust within the social structure of our world. The narcissist considers themselves as the epitome of uniqueness and that they should not have to mingle with ordinary rabble, or at the very least, those of lesser stature are unable to relate to them and understand them. Ultimately, the narcissist holds him or herself at an arm's length from people they deem below them, often objectifying these people and seeing them as instruments or tools to be used to meet their selfish ends.

- Another key aspect to narcissism, one we've already discussed, is that a narcissist must continuously receive affectations from the people they surround themselves with, if not from any individual. Admiration goes a long way for a narcissist due to the feeding and inflating of their ego, and upon finding a lack of admiration, that ego begins to deflate and the shell they built themselves starts to shrink back down to that small fragile self.

- Entitlement is a condition prevalent among many of the youth today, but it is also a trait key to narcissism. Narcissists not only believe the world should hand them their desires on a silver platter, they believe their every wish should be fulfilled. Queues? Who are those for? If any personality disorder was modeled after traditional monarchism, this would be it.

- Exploitation of others to achieve their goals, and upon satisfying those goals, the narcissist loses interest in the individual. This commonly takes place between the narcissist and those in close personal relationships with him or her, but is also present in smaller amounts among the narcissist and interactions with strangers. If a narcissist sees an opportunity to achieve one of their goals, or to gain something from the interaction, they will take it.

- Alongside exploitation, narcissists will commonly overlook the effects an action will have on others. A person can be easily cast aside by the narcissist, let alone any action taken that would leave the individual destitute in a manner of ways. Empathy is not a word narcissists relate to, and neither are the people they interact with. The narcissist can acknowledge what the other person is thinking of feeling, but they consider it of little consequence.

- Often a narcissist is weighing up those they encounter, whether it's in their circle of family and friends or colleagues and passersby, to see how they stack up alongside those individuals. This allows them to create a hierarchy in which they establish those they can and can't manipulate. If a narcissist encounters someone they believe is that much greater than them, they become envious. As a rule, most narcissists operate on the basis that those beneath them are jealous and envious of the narcissist, and that their reactions to narcissistic behavior and abuse stems out of this jealousy instead.

- Narcissists are often guilty of peacocking—that is, they behave in a grand and eye-catching manner. This often presents itself in arrogant and haughty overtures in the caricature of their behavior, often stilted and shallow, just another mask put on to satisfy their role.

The second method encompasses much of what has been covered in the above topics but the approach is drastically different. Instead of considering nine criteria, this model has broken it down into four groups within which an individual must exhibit impairment in their personality by showing characteristic difficulties in these groups.

These areas are identity of self, self-direction, empathy, and intimacy.

Both models corroborate that NPD always maintains the presence of grandiosity and attention-seeking behaviors.

While there are no particular physical characteristics that are clearly linked to NPD, many physical signs can show up from physical encounters as well as substance abuse. Most narcissists consume alcohol or drug substances to the extent that a physical toll is taken on their body.

The narcissist's mood, once examined, is often depressed. Polar to this mental state, once a narcissist is worked up into their grand displays, they can exhibit hypomania or mania—both being periods of hyperactive and excitable behavior, often paired with a short fuse, that impacts the regular machinations of day-to-day life. Hypomania is a milder version, rarely reaching the extent of manic highs, but also only lasting a couple of days at most. Mania is centered on a more present set of behavioral cues that last over a week. During this mania, narcissists are as likely to be fun as they are to lash out and hurt someone else; that is especially true if they were happy or anticipating happiness and it was taken away from them.

As mentioned before, it's plain to see that the rationality behind a narcissist's thoughts and behavior has sad roots. It helps us immensely to know the processes, however, in order to move forward. Now that we know the general background and neuroscience, we're going to discuss how to identify narcissists and catch those warning signs in action.

Self-Care

After narcissistic abuse, it's easy to forget about yourself. You might have been broken down to the point where you believe that you aren't worth caring about or you might think that the act of self-care is a form of vanity. No one who has suffered abuse at the hands of a narcissist wants to feel like one themselves, but that isn't what self-care is about.

The truth is, abuse or not, self-care is one of the most important things in anyone's life and most of us push it to one side, but now more than ever, you need to start putting yourself first. As indulgent as it might sound, self-care is vital for a healthy physical, emotional, and mental state. It's time for you to start rebuilding a happier relationship with yourself and self-care can help you do that for various reasons, including boosting your self-esteem and confidence, as well as increasing the production of positive feelings.

Of all the things that self-care can do for you, one of the most important is proving to yourself that you matter. You and your needs matter. This is something you need to not only remind yourself, but others. What better way to do that than to start following these healthy tips and steps to get to a better you? At the end of each chapter, we'll go over some healthy steps to recovering from the narcissistic patterns you've had to endure, all of which begin with self-care.

Step 1: Start a Journal

Some of the most memorable and influential people the world knows kept a journal, one of the most popular being Anne Frank. It kept a record of past events and the vivid memory of the writer, but one of the reasons those people kept writing was to feel the cathartic release of putting words and emotions down on paper. For most of us, speaking about our thoughts and the way we feel is a difficult feat. Pages don't judge us. They can't talk back and they can take everything we have to offer in a way very few people can ever do.

Journaling might seem strange and unfamiliar at first, but the more often you do it, the easier it becomes.

Here are some of the benefits of regularly freeing your mind by jotting it all down:

- Overthinking will slow down. Whenever you find yourself swimming—or drowning—in thoughts, you can start writing it all down instead. Allow the thoughts to leave you and slowly, you will find yourself resurfacing from beneath dark seas. It's important to leave the thoughts on the page. There's no use getting it all out if you are simply going to dive back into the deep end before you are ready.

- It resembles meditation in that you lose yourself to the act and afterwards, return to your life feeling relaxed because it's been shown to reduce stress. Find release in the act. Once it's all over, come back to yourself with renewed purpose.

- It makes you think and consider things you wouldn't ordinarily. The abstract becomes concrete, allowing for better understanding. With understanding comes the ability to move on rather than constantly questioning everything. It's a great way to resolve arguments or solve problems. You'll get to know yourself better too.

- You might find yourself becoming more creative with each word you put down. Writing helps us process things more efficiently. This can lead to new opportunities, interesting webs of thoughts, and unlocking memories you never knew you had.

Keeping a journal might be difficult if you've never done it before. The key is to keep writing; you will get better at it the more you do it. Various studies have shown that journaling, specifically about thoughts, emotions, *and* feelings, rather than only one of the three, has helped many people who suffer from illness, mental disorders, and past abuse and trauma (Pennebaker, 2014). The physical and mental health benefits are well-known.

Don't worry about where you will find the time for journaling either. As with everything, if you make it a priority, you will definitely find time for it. It doesn't have to be long; one 10-15 minute session out of your day is more than enough to reap the benefits.

You have 10-15 minutes a day to spare, don't you?

Chapter 2.

The Depths of Narcissism; A Look at the Types and Subtypes

Due to the complexity of narcissism, and the burgeoning understandings that are brought to light with every new case study, several archetypes have been laid out under the general category of narcissism. Upon encountering a new situation, especially in which survival instincts are triggered, the brain tries to restructure itself to handle the new situation—a compromise is often struck, creating a similar, but not exactly the same, circumstance.

Psychologists and researchers have dug into the depths of narcissism to better understand the condition and its various iterations. Narcissism, like any mental disorder, has many faces and any one of these can appear in your everyday life. It's a great step that you've taken to finding solace in the understanding of narcissism and the toolset you've acquired in the first chapter, however there is more to narcissism than lies in flamboyance and manipulation.

The narcissistic traits mentioned prior are tied directly to narcissism as a general study under which there are several subtypes. In order to properly defend against a narcissist, especially the more extreme variations, it is essential to know what they are and what drives them to behave in the manner they do. There are three main types, as well as several subtypes that can be applied to the main types—beyond that there are two special extreme subtypes, one of which is narcissism that depends on the cycle of abuse provided by other narcissists.

Breaking down the various facets of narcissism, you will come to see that while generally after the same concepts, each narcissistic profile operates differently. The common trope used to portray the narcissist in most Western media specifically fits the overt and grandiose archetype. Most people will have come to familiarize themselves with at least the appearance and some basic traits of the narcissist through these external influences, but it is only a fraction of the totality of narcissism. To treat every narcissist as if they were this particular archetype could cause more damage within the dynamic held between the two of you. A malignant or sadistic narcissist may respond violently if challenged in the same manner as an overt narcissist would be treated.

Don't worry if those terms aren't gaining purchase right now, they didn't mean much to me when I first heard about them, but as I started dealing with more trouble in my life, I had to look at the depths of narcissism. I'm here to explain to you what those terms mean, what those narcissists look like, and how to identify them. Understanding and identification comes before healing as you are dealing with the immediate situation to stop further wounding. This acts like emergency response care and will help to stem the flow of blood from the earlier wounds that have been inflicted, and after that comes a time for proper treatment and care.

Together we are going to plumb the depths of narcissism and uncover all the dirty secrets they try to hide from you. It's not always a pretty sight but that is the truth of the abuse behind narcissism—-on the surface it can be all superb and finery, but under the surface is a festering wound. Like any wound, as soon as you start looking for the evidence guided by the correct signs, you will find it in no time.

The warning signs of narcissistic abuse will help you protect yourself against the narcissists in your life before you get caught in their trap. We will cover warning signs that will act as red flags for any person you engage with. Narcissists are opportunists at heart and may strike at any time, honeyed words and sincerity that are entirely a falsehood.

Let's take a look at the specialties that narcissistic personality disorder has accrued under its banner and the truth behind the individuals suffering from that subtype.

Profiling the Narcissist

Perhaps the hardest part about figuring out whether someone is a narcissist is that there is no definitive test. No blood test or scan is going to reveal that a person is a narcissist. Instead, psychologists determine this by observation and psychological evaluations. They'll identify certain character traits, changes in attitude, patterns of behavior, and types of reactions in order to gauge their patient.

At first glance, this might seem like a difficult thing to do, especially if you aren't an experienced therapist, but that isn't the case. It's actually easier than you think, quite simply because narcissistic symptoms are right in front of our eyes. Odds are you know exactly what a narcissist is, but you've overlooked the patterns that point to this conclusion. Nevertheless, we've all encountered that one guy who always turns the conversation around so you are talking about him or that one lady who thinks she's better than you will ever be. The disorder comes in different shapes and sizes and it's best to avoid them at all costs. Most of the time, narcissists are charismatic to a fault, luring people in with generosity and false friendliness. This is confusing because it gives you the sense that they might actually be nice. That would be easier to believe than that a person could be self-centered and lacking in compassion.

Inviting them into your life would be much like inviting a vampire to step over the threshold of your house—an energy vampire, that is. Since there are so many, it's important to know which is which and how to keep them away from you. There's a theory that states the best way to find out if a narcissist is a narcissist is to simply ask them if they are. The experiment relies on the idea that narcissists, having no shame about the way they are, they might tell the truth. Indeed, they might even be proud of it.

Types of Narcissists

There are three main types of narcissists, each categorized by their own sub-types. These are the classic narcissist, the vulnerable narcissist, and the malignant narcissist. The importance of knowing the differences comes in when one tries to react or get away from the narcissist. If dealing with the malignant narcissist, for example, one would not be able to use the same methods as they would with a vulnerable narcissist. The way they function is not the same and misunderstanding this can lead to feelings of uncertainty.

Perhaps they aren't really a narcissist after all, just because they don't exhibit the behavior I've read about. Perhaps we can overcome this. Perhaps I'm reading too much into things.

Perhaps they're telling the truth instead of making excuses. Perhaps there's room for hope that they'll change.

These are all questions that you can find yourself asking. They're questions I asked myself and it wasn't until I found out that there was more than one kind that I realized just how much information I had missing from my arsenal, that I wasn't wrong about the narcissists I'd come across in my lifetime, both blood-relatives and otherwise, but instead that I didn't realize what exactly I was dealing with. Things are already confusing once you find out about the narcissist in your life or once you begin to suspect there is one, and even more so if they're manipulating you or acting like two different people. You don't know where or how you stand. Consider this information a set of tools to cope and recover. I'm giving you some new tools that will help you identify and escape from the torments of narcissism. Without further ado, let's find out more about the different types of narcissists.

- Classic: As the name suggests, this is the narcissist we all know about. They're the ones who seek attention and boast about every tiny achievement. They want you to flatter them, admire them, and shower them with affection. If you don't give in to the worship they feel entitled to, they're likely to become distant and bored. They look down on almost everyone and yet, they feed on praise from others. These are the greedy, grandiose, overconfident narcissists.

- Vulnerable: Nearly the polar opposite of the classic type, the vulnerable narcissist hates having the spotlight shone on them. They're also known as victim and closet narcissists for this reason. They still have the same superiority complex as a classic narcissist, but they usually get their desired quota of attention by seeking pity and/or acting generous.

They're normally found on the arm of someone special or successful; special or successful by association rather than chasing the treatment for themselves.

- Malignant: When you hear about narcissistic abuse, this is usually where it all starts. This type is also known as the toxic narcissist. They're sadistic in a way that separates them from the other two types, manipulative and exploitative. Deceit and aggression are usually the way forward for this type and, as we spoke about above, they lack any remorse. Without empathy and a commonly found sadistic streak, this narcissist potentially enjoys making others suffer and has even been compared to sociopaths and psychopaths.

- Subtype 1: Overt and covert. Their names are fairly self-explanatory. Covert narcissists work under the cover of subtle and passive-aggressive action. They're harder to catch at their game. This is one of the most common subtypes in narcissistic abuse because they're stealthy in that they leave their victims feeling confused and anyone on the outside can find it difficult to believe there was any abuse at all. On the other hand, overt narcissists will boast and insult openly and unmistakably.

  o The vulnerable type is always covert.

  o The classic type is always overt.

  o Meanwhile, the malignant type can be either.

- Subtype 2: Somatic and cerebral. This is all down to what the narcissist values in themselves and in others. For instance, somatic narcissists are some of the common ones we hear about in that they are obsessed with their own physical appearance, vain, and often found in the gym or splurging on an insane skin/hair care range. Cerebral narcissists are much the same; the only difference is that they're concentrated more on their academic and intellectual prowess. They believe themselves to be the smartest in the room rather than the most externally attractive. Any of the three main types can fall into these subtypes depending on their mode of gain; using their bodies as deceptive tools or using their accomplishments as methods of attention-seeking, among other things.

- Special Subtypes: Inverted and sadistic. Research sometimes brings up rarer cases of narcissists. These fall into "special" subtypes—but don't let the narcissist think they're special; it's not like they need the ego boost.

  o Inverted narcissists are believed to also be the covert vulnerable type. They're codependent, clinging specifically onto other narcissists to feel special and understood. Generally, they show signs of abandonment issues, often from childhood, and their victim-nature leaves them feeling unsatisfied unless they are in relationships with people like themselves, namely the other narcissists.

  o Sadistic narcissists are the ones who resemble sociopaths and psychopaths in that they derive pleasure from the pain of others. They're malignant, aggressive, and controlling. This normally extends into their sex lives as their desire to hurt and humiliate people is in line with several existing fetishes.

45

Spotting Narcissists by the Classic Signs of Narcissism

You have learnt about the various aspects of what makes a narcissist tick, but their deplorable behavior is not only limited to that. Narcissistic personality disorder will always be coupled with a cycle of abuse when the narcissist has someone they can prey upon and that abuse is always specifically geared to the outcome the narcissist desires.

This behavior is often systematic, and it will carry the same telltale signs as any other abuse in narcissistic relationships. Familiarizing you with this cycle, as well as the intent behind the actions of the narcissist, will create an environment in which it is easier to dodge the mines laid out by the narcissist.

- Nobody is better at a first impression than a narcissist. You will be positively blown away by their personality while simultaneously being left without a bad word to remark on them. In this time, the narcissist does everything right, going out of their way to see to your every whim. This period lasts, but only for a short while before it's the narcissist who has flipped the script and is trying to play your role while forcing you to run around after them.

- Narcissists will often drive the topic of conversation, particularly steering it in their own direction—about themselves, of course—and leaving little room for anyone else to enter into the conversation. This is often out of a desire to appear self-assured, especially if that's the last thing the narcissist is feeling. Narcissists domineer the conversation in this manner because they believe they are above everyone else, sneering down from on high, and in doing so will often refuse to engage in a conversational topic that is not about them or can't be redirected back to them.

- Narcissists find comfort in the praise of others. A narcissist cannot support their personality from within and so they search outside of themselves, in other people, to find a sense of worthiness. Acceptance, validation, and praise are what a narcissist most wants out of any human engagement and if they're not receiving the attention they feel they deserve, they will start pushing buttons until they get it, or at least a reaction of some kind.

- Lasting relationships can be a sore point for a narcissist, mostly because the narcissist is as likely to chase the other individual away as they are to dump them in the dust and find the latest model on the market. The lack of empathy evident within narcissism plays a crucial factor in this as the narcissist engages with the individual only on the terms of their own needs and desires, but they fail to consider what the desires of the individual are, and whether or not the narcissist's outcomes and that of the individual are conflicting.

- Narcissists are mean. This isn't the stereotypical put down of a cranky colleague at work, but rather a statement made to cut. The importance of the subject they are degrading you for is less important than the fact that they can spin that target around and use it as ammunition against you. The malignant obsession of a narcissist to bring others down will become pervasive and quickly evident as you spend time with them.

- Given the behavior linked to interpersonal compliments and long-term relationships, it is no surprise that narcissists often have difficulty settling on a label or term for their current relationship. No clear term will be applied to the relationship for the narcissist—often they are simply there to collect the emotional benefits and rewards of a committed relationship, but keeping a loose connection to the relationship allows them a method to satisfy that need currently but alongside the freedom to leave if a better, worthier prospect comes up.

- As much as a narcissist loves to use their words to twist and turn you this way and that, a narcissist will use double-speak to create an entirely new narrative for the same argument you've been having. Often, a narcissist will use this double-speak to bull over you and impress a new recollection of the situation on you, painting you as the perpetrator and they as they victim.

- Narcissism is centered around the belief that one is special, a cut above the rest, and this belief will place a strain on any relationship when the narcissist is at fault. First, they will deny any wrongdoing and refuse to accept responsibility or blame for the actions they took or the words they said. They refuse to believe they could be incorrect or at fault, and even once it has been pointed out to the narcissist with undeniable fact that they were the cause, no apology will be forthcoming.

- When you try to leave a relationship with a narcissist, they will begin to panic. For the entirety of your relationship, you have been the fuel that was sustaining the narcissist while burning away at yourself. A narcissist will stop at nothing to hold on to you and they may begin by doing everything correctly, showering you with affection and love-bombs, but it can take on a sinister edge under the guise of blackmail and threats. Removing a narcissist's claws from your flesh can be painful in of itself but it is a necessary step to shedding the influence and trauma caused by their abuse.

- A narcissist is a storyteller at heart, and they will inundate you with the dullest of tales at your merest behest, and you can use this trait to your favor. A narcissist's tale centers around themselves and reflects only on that experience, and so a success story that involved the narcissist becomes impossible without their involvement, regardless of their actual contribution. Additionally, in any tale that goes awry, a narcissist will refuse to take on any form of blame. There is no possibility for them to be found at fault, at least in their minds, and they will stubbornly maintain that storyline.

Self-Care

The thing about abuse is that it messes up the normal processes in the brain. For the most part, people with mental disorders are born with them. There are times, however, where mental disorders can be developed based on external factors such as the environment and climate we were raised in. When it comes to abuse victims, the brain can literally rewire itself. The chemicals it produces can be negatively affected by a broken down self-esteem, a lack of confidence, and the nagging feelings and sensations instilled into it by the abuser.

Step 2: Meditate

There are ways to cope with the crippling weight of toxicity and overcome the sense of blame and guilt we experience even when we aren't the ones in the wrong. One such way is meditation. We all know this is a trending topic, but what exactly are the benefits that have everyone jumping onto the daily meditation bandwagon?

Apart from the obvious reason, that being that it's actually a really enjoyable practice, there are several health benefits to meditating on a regular basis:

- Our first action step to self-care and recovery was to journal. Meditation can actually improve this process, if indirectly. This is because it's been proven to improve our concentration, which in turn allows us to become better at creative pursuits including writing.

- It helps turn the mountains back into molehills. One of the things meditation does is turn you into a more self-aware person and with self-awareness comes the realization that now is all that really matters. By meditating often, you will find your brain rewiring itself to follow more positive patterns and one such positive change will be the ability to stop worrying about the past or the future by detaching from meaningless things and focusing more on the bigger picture—the present.

- Meditation has been proven to alleviate stress and anxiety. It reduces blood pressure and improves the heart's condition. Why wouldn't you want to start improving your physical health *and* your mental health?

- It's true that enlightenment is a term often heard by people who practice meditation regularly. Did you know that enlightenment isn't something that comes from the outside, but rather something that comes from within? Meditation forces you to look within yourself, to allow your thoughts and feelings to pass with acknowledgement rather than obsession, and to understand yourself on a deeper level. It's this enlightenment that could be what helps you find your purpose in life and if not that, you might just find a version of yourself you either didn't know existed or thought you had lost a long time ago.

- Though the narcissists in our lives are the bad guy we're aiming to conquer, each of us has demons of our own. Some people use meditation to overcome specific thoughts, emotions, and behaviors, especially those which are unhealthy. While smoking or drinking are typical things to stop doing, you might find small tendencies you'd like to rid yourself of, certainly tendencies that you feel could have contributed to the abuse experienced. Never blame yourself for the abuse, but remember that we are not all perfect. One of the crucial steps to recovery is to take responsibility for your own involvement or antagonization in the relationship between yourself and the narcissist.

As with journaling, if you want to meditate, it will take dedication and prioritization. You need to make the time. You'll also need to practice because it won't be easy at first. In fact, sometimes new meditators are unable to manage more than five minutes. Don't give up and you will find yourself lasting longer and reaping more benefits with each session.

Find a place where you won't be disturbed, make sure you are comfortably sitting or lying down, and ensure that there is peace and quiet whenever you meditate. It's recommended to try out some audiobooks or online videos and follow their instructions. Don't eat before you meditate, or you will end up feeling lethargic.

Why would that be bad, you ask? Lethargy creates a feeling of fatigue and meditation often requires you to concentrate on one thing at a time in an effort to declutter the mind, and lethargy can lead your mind to distraction, or fully into slumber. The idea is to teach your mind to concentrate on one thing in order to let go of everything else. This method will move over into your day-to-day life, preventing you from concentrating on lingering thoughts and instead letting them pass you by like the clouds in the sky with each deep breath that you take.

Chapter 3.

Learn to Stand Up for Yourself in the Face of Narcissism and Gaslighting

The dreaded emotional abuse upon which narcissists and gaslighters heavily rely on can both be precursors to physical abuse. Even though it can fly under the radar, mental and emotional abuse are just as dangerous. It can leave lasting damage on one's mental health to the extent that they might suffer from PTSD.

What do you do when you find yourself stuck in this pattern? First of all, know that you are not alone and the abuse is not something that you deserve. No one deserves any form of abuse. Secondly, note that it is going to take time to recover and that recovery is extremely possible.

Below are some ways you can start the process of recovery, by handing yourself and your trust over to other people:

- Seek out professional help. While it is possible to heal and recover on your own, there's really no need to reject or refuse help when it is so easily available to you. I understand that it may be difficult to reach out—it's a brave step and one not taken without great deliberation. The impact emotional and psychological abuse have can make you think that seeing a therapist is a sign of weakness or mental instability. In actuality, many are trained specifically to help survivors of abuse and with that experience, they will make it easier for you to start transforming your mental and emotional processes into healthier ones.

- If you aren't comfortable with seeking out help in person, try a text or telephonic option. There are various helplines that are open 24/7 and easy for you to reach. It might be easier to confront another human with the way you are feeling and the things you are going through if you don't have to bear your soul to a stranger sitting in front of you. The anonymity of text and telephone lines can provide a safety net. Once you've grown in confidence and taken a few more steps toward healing, you may feel better about approaching someone in reality.

- Sometimes, professional help isn't the only help out there. If you've been trapped in an abusive cycle, it's highly likely that most, if not all of the people you used to rely on are no longer around. A method of controlling the victim is to isolate them, meaning that the abuser either gets your friends and family to turn on you or gets you to turn on them. This can make things harder than ever because having people in your corner is always helpful. That's what motivates boxers and wrestlers in the ring, right? They have someone there to push them through it, hand them the water, and pull them back when they think it's reaching breaking point. It's difficult to rebuild our lives after abuse and it can be stressful and overwhelming. Don't focus on all the big fears that you have on your shoulders. Instead, start small by doing something like joining a club or going to a yoga class or reaching out to those people who really matter to you. The least you can do is try, right? If you are rejected, you can still say that you put yourself out there and rather than give up, you can move onto the next option. There are plenty of those available to you. All you have to do is dig deep, find the courage, and reach out to grab them.

Shift Your Perspective

Unless it's consensual and happens behind closed doors, there should be no power-play in your relationships. The second someone starts trying to control you or your life, you should probably run as far as you can in the opposite direction. Unfortunately, however, this isn't always an option. As much as we hate to admit it, there are times where we simply can't cut off contact with the narcissists in our lives. They could be family members, colleagues, or even the parents of your children. Whatever the relationship, it's safe to say that cutting narcissists off, while preferable, is not always the only way to deal with them.

I'd highly recommend that you do engage in no contact if you can, but if not, let's look at how you can start standing up for yourself and setting healthy boundaries to take back control of your own life.

You need to start viewing yourself as a survivor instead of a victim. This is the first step to change—changing the perspective you have of yourself after abuse. It's time to start building new foundations.

If you are this far into this book, you are already on your way to repairing the damage, restoring your self-worth, and regaining confidence lost to your abuser. Everything you've learned so far has increased your knowledge and awareness, which are key to growing your sense of self. At this point, it's up to you to turn to yourself for the clarity you once sought from your abuser. Don't worry, I'll guide you through it.

Whatever obligations force you to keep narcissists in your life, it's important not to let them control you. In plain terms, this is a no-bullshit list to help you keep your defenses up and maintain rationality in these interactions. You have to honor your own needs most.

Keep Your Expectations Low

You should go into interactions with narcissists expecting nothing. It's good to appreciate the good because, let's face it, you *can* have good times with a narcissist, but you need to leave it there. The bad can come out at any moment and you need to practice self-protection and emotional detachment to avoid getting hurt. Use the tips on this list to keep those guards up.

They Aren't Going to Change

It's true that people can change, but when it comes to narcissists, that hardly ever happens. The way their brains function prevents them from understanding the effects they have on other people. To an extent, they even believe that there's nothing wrong with the way they act and that it's other people who have the problem.

Without actually addressing their behavior, or recognizing and acknowledging it at all, they can't change. The lack of empathy and responsibility can make someone like you, a compassionate person by nature, lose your mind. Instead of going crazy over something you can't control, let go and realize that they are incapable on a fundamental level to change and it's up to you to change your own reactions and interactions because they're all you really can control.

Don't Engage or Let Yourself Get Dragged into an Argument

You can still be polite without revealing too much about yourself. By keeping the information you share to a minimum, you will find it much easier to avoid conflict. Narcissists look down on their victims, but if you leave them with mere surface details, it'll be harder for them to latch onto you. Personal information will be used against you. Beware of how much fuel you choose to give an arsonist.

With the knowledge that they won't change, you can win every fight with a narcissist by simply refusing to get into one. Don't take the bait, respond blandly, and give nothing solid. Change the subject, evade it, or leave them with a lack of agreement or disagreement on your end.

Eventually, they'll get bored and leave you alone.

Don't Take Anything Personally

This goes along with the previous item on the list, but from a different angle, think not about what releasing expectations will do in terms of the narcissist and instead what it will do in terms of your own mental and emotional state. What the narcissist does has nothing to do with you and everything to do with themselves. You have no reason to let the guilt-trips get to you.

Once you realize this, you will have added an extra layer of emotional protection to help you set up boundaries.

Don't Be Afraid to Withdraw When You've Had Enough

If things become too much, you feel you can no longer be positive, or you think it's getting too negative for you to handle, remove yourself from the situation. Self-preservation is the only way to put a stop to abuse because ultimately, it's up to you to protect your emotions and mental state. Don't let anyone dictate the importance of your engagement in a conversation.

You never have to remain near a person who makes you uncomfortable in the slightest manner.

Take Company with You

Remind yourself that you are not alone. Take a witness with you, someone who can be a rational audience to the narcissist without getting drawn in by the things they say—particularly if they are negative and about you. Narcissists like to ruin the reputation of their victims, but if you take someone with an objective point of view or someone the narcissist will behave around, you save yourself from the type of behavioral patterns they would normally exhibit when the two of you are alone.

Bear in mind that narcissists don't usually mind saying or doing harmful things in public spaces, but their tactics include making their victim look insane. It's harder to deny their actions when there are witnesses around. In this case, you will finally have the upper hand in the situation.

You can even come up with safety words or cues with the person you choose to help you out of an uncomfortable situation. For example, when you feel that it's time to withdraw from the situation and you aren't sure how to do it, a signal will call that person over to you. Just like that, you've got yourself an easy out that the narcissist cannot prevent without putting themselves at risk.

Appreciate the Healthy Relationships in Your Life

Earlier in the book, we discussed how the people who surround narcissists also suffer and that those with mental disorders tend to be treated with more importance. Similarly, you have to acknowledge that your own trauma and history of abuse can affect those around you. It's hard not to get caught up in toxic cycles when they happen to the people we love.

It's because of this that you need to take the time to thank the people in your life who can help you through the healing process. You will get through this together. Make sure they know that they're appreciated and do your very best not to take anything you are experiencing out on them.

Be Proud of Yourself for Your Progress

The mere fact that you are *trying* to improve your life, your health, and your relationships shows courage. It's not an easy thing to do, especially when so many of the steps require personal strength and growth. Once you discover that it's really up to you to heal, it can seem easier to turn away from the process. It's a tough journey, but one well worth sticking out.

Though you will likely have several people who love and care for you to help you through healing, most of the battles you have to go through are internal. They involve self-care and self-nurturing; two things we might sometimes feel we don't deserve or have time for. No matter what happens, it's crucial that you reward yourself for getting through it and for withdrawing as you need to.

No one knows what's best for you but you and so, it's up to you to make sure those lines are in place and no one crosses them without your say.

Self-Care

To get straight to the point: you need to learn how to say no. There are people in this world who are going to try and walk all over you and you have to do your best not to let them. Put your foot down and let go of the fear of letting others down. Think to yourself, when you reflexively agree or allow this behavior to continue, are you letting *yourself* down?

You matter more than that. You deserve better, so maybe you should start giving yourself better before you start trying to obtain it from others. You have to stop falling for the traps and start setting up some boundaries.

Step 3: Set Clear Boundaries

Hours spent worrying about how to stick to or how to get out of impossible promises can leave you stressed and drained. Don't undermine your own efforts to improve your life by prioritizing others first. Stop the cycle before your energy is completely depleted and take a few steps back to assess the situation.

Some tips for saying no:

- Take time. Don't immediately agree. Instead, say something like, "I'll think about it and get back to you." This way, you will have more time to process the request, whether you want to or can do it, and how the end result will make you feel. You'll be more sure of your answer and therefore be able to say no with more gusto.

- Don't confuse refusal with rejection. People generally understand that you are allowed to say no as much as they are allowed to ask you something. It's universally agreed upon that you should prepare for either answer when asking for a favor rather than expecting a confirmation.

- Compromise. Only do this is if the request is actually something you want to agree to. Never allow yourself to be pressured. Suggest a way for the request to suit both of you. If you really want to or need to say no, don't suggest a compromise.

- Keep it simple. Use firm and direct phrases without necessarily saying no as this could be a trigger. An example would be, "Thanks for coming to me, but unfortunately I'm not able to help out at this time." Don't apologize further than that. You have no reason to ask permission to refuse and certainly no reason to feel guilty for it.

- Be true to you. The more you get to know yourself through these steps, the better you will become at examining yourself. You have to be honest and clear about what you really want.

Chapter 4.

Take a Step into Reality and Start Writing Your Own Story

It is common knowledge that the narcissist is preoccupied with delusions of self-grandeur, but the delusions don't stop there. Much like any person, a narcissist will preoccupy themselves with daydreams in spare moments, but the fervor and intent behind the dream is exceptionally different.

A normal daydream is mostly filler and fluffy clouds and blissful ignorance, but for a narcissist it is the spoils of war. These daydreams are often filled with a variety of imagery that depicts themselves as dominant, successful, influential, and conquering—the content often surrounding hostile events, sexual content, dreams of what they expect the future to be, and self-revealing.

It is often these stories that the narcissist utilizes to reinforce their ego, especially when they are depleting their narcissistic supply (the extent of the narcissist's validation accrued from others) and they are unable to use someone to gain their artificial reinforcement, they turn introspective and begin to fantasize. It is in this that the narcissist and the ordinary person differ, as the narcissist is floundering inside an emptiness they can't explain, panic-stricken.

Once inside these fantasies, a narcissist can become severely lost and disoriented within their identity, often seeking a cold comfort, if any, and using it to shape their reality. A narcissist will choose to remain in a position of suffering and self-loathing because they have become accustomed to that state and now have found it reasonably assured. It is safe, if not pleasurable.

Certainty and control, or the lack thereof, plays a role in the narcissist's sense of grandeur—to be assured of what would occur in their future, the narcissist would choose a secure but uncomfortable position to maintain that feeling of justification and value. It seems almost as if there is an emptiness or an incapability within the narcissist to produce self-value and they remain on a rollercoaster of chasing acknowledgment and running from panic.

The Fantasy of Expectations

While this fantasy doesn't strictly remain in the narcissist's head, they certainly expect you to be able to see in there to figure out what they expect from you. Unfortunately, narcissists are exceptionally demanding in their expectations while remaining unsympathetic to an individual's needs; the only thing that is relevant is what the narcissist wants and that you haven't done it yet. A narcissistic partner is often so preoccupied with themselves that when it comes to their needs, they don't process the reality that you haven't spent the last hour figuring out what exactly your narcissist needs today.

Alongside the unrealistic demand that you pluck the very thought from their gray matter, a narcissist's fuse is often unrealistically short which often leads to bristly engagements over petty decisions that will mean nothing within the next hour, let alone the next month or year. Pressing the narcissist onto the defensive here would create a troublesome space as this can provoke unpredictable tantrums, episodes of "as-ifs," a feeling of indignation presented at imagined slights, false accusations, and even violent behavior.

The Reality of the Narcissist's Vulnerability

It is the narcissist's own outrageous belief in themselves that creates such a fragile and shaky identity—a narcissist has faith in their own omnipotence. They are untouchable, indestructible, and glorious above us all. Despite the ironbound conviction, it simply isn't true, and once a narcissist has been presented with an indisputable reconciliation of their personal claim, the narcissist becomes bristly and enraged, unable to withstand the affront to their personal beliefs.

While narcissists can dish out punishment in the form of degrading commentary, any challenge that is made to the structure of the narcissist's false self-identity is met with scorn and rage. It is the understanding of the narcissist that the only object holding them back from achievement of any particular form is simply their volition. The self-assured nature of the narcissist presents itself when the narcissist is confident that whatever their will, it shall be, and it merely depends on gathering their will to see it accomplished. The option to fail is not conceived in the mind of the narcissist.

This creates a division between the narcissist and reality, and in doing so, a warped perspective is created within the narcissist that cannot reconcile the truth of their own worth and abilities. This further feeds the need for a narcissistic supply and an external support as the idea of their self-worth becomes damaged and warped to a point it is unrecognizable.

Rewrite Your Life

As you can see, the stories that we tell ourselves can be beneficial in that they bolster us against the storm of life, but they can, too, become a devastating weapon that we create and turn against ourselves. The voice in your head is exceptionally powerful, not only because of its proximity to you but also due to its familiarity. You will believe what you tell yourself, no matter if that particular item is good or bad.

Your voice is your most powerful tool, and the narcissist knows this, and so they will do what they can to limit your voice and influence in any engagements with them, but furthermore, they will try to sow doubt in your mind about your choices, your opinions, and in your intelligence. Narcissists are cruel and vindictive, and they only see defaming you as a tool to expedite their desired outcome, instead of any of the damage and repercussions they are afflicting you with.

The reality is that you hold a tenuous position in your own life—you are your decision maker and that allows you to be your own hero, or to become your greatest nemesis. You get the option to rewrite your life's story; you no longer have to play the victim role to satisfy the needs of someone else.

You have come a long way already on your journey to independence and healing and this would be the perfect time to ground yourself in your reality, the one you deserve, before we head on to discuss how to heal from the damage caused by narcissistic personality disorder.

To do that we are going to call on some of the self-care tools you've picked up on so far: journaling and saying no. Get out your journal and start listing important aspects in your life. This should include your career, your family, your hobbies and friends, but also negative aspects such as narcissists in your life if they're not already listed. You want a pretty thorough list so that you can create a clearer picture of what to keep and what to remove from your life.

Once you've finalized your list, go back through it and consider which aspects of your life affect you the most and why. Circle the most important parts of your life that are good for you; this is where you can focus your efforts to get your confidence back.

The negatives aren't getting left out—you are kicking them out. Figure out what detractors in your life are taking the biggest toll, and circle them as well. I'm fairly certain your narcissist is one of the items on that list now. The objective with your negative items is to either change them to a beneficial prospect, or to get rid of it entirely. However, you are now armed with focus.

Finally, after setting your goals and your boundaries, it's time for you to consider what you want for your own life. The next chapter will guide you through healing from the emotional and mental trauma that narcissistic abuse places on an individual. It will help you to free yourself of that burden and change the landscape of your future entirely.

Self-Care

Particularly, when you are preoccupied with the negative emotions going through you from being trapped in a negative and traumatic environment, it can be easy to forget what it's like to simply do something for fun. When was the last time you did something you actually love? This step of self-care is all about finding that one thing you used to do or finding something new to do for the simple sake of enjoyment.

Step 4: Take Up a Hobby

Hobbies are not just for people who have a lot of time on their hands. They have numerous health benefits, exactly like the other steps we've already covered. Here are a few:

- Engaging in activities we enjoy in our free time improve the mind and body. Depression and anxiety are reduced and so are blood pressure and total cortisol, among other things. It's the perfect step to a healthier you.

- They reduce stress. When you lose yourself to an act that you enjoy, focusing on having fun rather than work or the negative things plaguing you, you will notice all your stresses fade away. Having fun instead of worrying will help you focus on the present moment and the things you love doing.

- Taking breaks are some of the most important things you can do for yourself and hobbies give you that option whilst still doing something. Some people struggle to take breaks because they feel unproductive. With hobbies, you can take breaks and have fun with a sense of purpose.

- Meeting new people can come from finding hobbies. Of course, it's important to keep your walls up and remember the things you've learned about narcissists and gaslighting so far, but connecting with people who enjoy and feel passionate about the same things you do can be refreshing and exciting. Don't close yourself off to the idea of meeting like-minded people because of your past experiences.

- Hobbies promote eustress, a positive type of stress. It's that rush of excitement and happiness that you may be familiar with. Doing something you love is the perfect way to unlock that type of stress.

Keep an open mind because finding your hobby won't always be easy. It has to come naturally for it to last—you can't force yourself to just like something. Try new things, especially if your friends are doing them, because you never know what your next pastime is going to be!

Chapter 5.

Getting a Grip on Life

You've made it this far and you are doing so well. By now you've struck the shackles from your wrists that narcissistic abuse had placed on you and you are well on your way to becoming yourself.

Now that you've escaped the cycle of abuse and your wounds are beginning to close, it's time to start a new chapter in your life, one that may be fraught with misadventure and mayhem but definitely not one torn apart by pathological narcissism.

The cycle you were trapped in was a dark one without much hope for a future that was different, and lost in that world you likely lost sight of your future and what is important to you. The first step on the next leg of your journey is to envision what you want out of life. If you aren't making your own decisions and your own plans, making the best use of your time, someone else will come along and try and make those decisions for you and take that time away from you.

It is important to have a clear vision of the goals and achievements you are setting out to achieve; otherwise, you will get lost in the daily monotony, and months and years pass with little progress.

Get together some writing materials to create a few lists. Each list will focus on your goals, your desires, and your aspirations over different time periods. Create a list each for the short term, the medium term, and long term goals.

On your paper, for your long term goals, consider writing where you want to be and what you want to achieve in over ten years from now. Also, consider the things you would most like to say you have achieved in your life and add this to this portion of the lists.

Now on to your list for your medium term goals, these goals would be expected to take place sometime within the next five years. These goals are likely larger goals that will take some time or doing to achieve, but they are important goals that are accessible to you.

And finally, your third list will come together forming your immediate goals. These you can complete with little to no effort within the next year. Some of these items should include steps that will take you toward your middle and long term goals.

Now for each of your lists, you are going to go over the items again but highlight a handful out of each list. For your long term and major goals, I'd recommend only selecting one or two goals and setting that as your initial achievement off of that list, moving on to the next once you have completed the first. On your medium and short term lists, I recommend picking no more than five per each list, with the same mindset applied where you replace a completed goal with your next most important.

This creates a simple but structured overview of what you want out of life; you've done away with any distractions from your true goals and you will be able to work toward fulfilling them without being pulled in a thousand directions. You now can guide yourself through life and make informed decisions when it comes to the tough choices in your life.

The Trap Hanging Open Above You at All Times

Now that you've escaped your abuse and the atrocities they made you suffer through, you have gained an immense amount of freedom. It is all too easy for someone who has gone through this abuse to slip straight back into the cycle. Narcissist's are oily socializers, and before you know it, they're talking you right back into accepting their abuse.

Don't stand for it. Refuse to take their garbage and turn your attention elsewhere. It is a good idea to keep your support updated on when the narcissist contacts you or at least tries to. Your support network will be the main safety net keeping you out of the narcissist's arms and from running back to them.

In each of these instances, it is best to maintain a strong support network to find the best results. Fighting against a narcissist and recurring narcissistic abuse is a long and often lonely road, and sometimes a friendly face is the only thing that will get you through to the next day.

Self-Care

As humans, we are all prone to overthinking things now and then. The problem comes in when overthinking becomes your default setting. It can bring up bad memories, negative words, and terrible images.

Two destructive thought patterns can come from overthinking, neither of which are good for your soul or mood: worrying and ruminating. Spending too much time focusing on the negative, dwelling on the past, and persistent worrying can all be catastrophic to your daily life. You might find yourself unable to get anything done and with elevated stress levels and clouded judgment, you might not want to make any more to act at all.

Step 5: Stop Overthinking

Before you can tackle this habit, you need to actively make yourself aware of it. If ever you find yourself doubting, take a step back and look at the situation from an outside perspective. If the way you are responding is unnecessarily anxious or uncalled for, use this seed of awareness to gauge any moment of overthinking and then you can proceed to put a stop to it and make the changes you want to make.

Here's how:

- Put a timer on it. It's not easy to simply stop overthinking, but if you give yourself a boundary of 5-10 minutes to simply worry and analyze everything, you get it out of your system. You might even want to write it all down and throw it away once time runs out. After that, you can turn to more positive methods of passing time.

- Gain some perspective. An easy way to stop your thoughts in their tracks is to ask yourself how much they will matter in a few years or even a few weeks' time. Thinking about the bigger picture and switching up the time frame can help turn off the thoughts.

- Make an effort to learn about and practice mindfulness. This one goes along with meditation. It's all about breathing and focusing on the present moment. Mindfulness takes practice, but with time and effort, you will notice your overthinking tendencies start to fade away.

- Challenge your thoughts. Emotions can mess with our ability to look at things in an objective manner. Gather all the evidence you can that prove your thoughts are or aren't true before you make the split-second decision to act on them or let them overtake you.

- Solve problems. It isn't helpful to dwell on problems, but it is to look for solutions to them. If the problem is something you have control over, you can make an effort to prevent or challenge it. Give yourself the task of identifying it and then put in the effort to come up with at least five possible ways to resolve it. If it's not something you have control over, you have to focus on the way you handle and cope with it instead. The change starts with your attitude.

The mind is a muscle and needs to be trained to change. Over time, building healthier habits will help you grow mentally stronger. As with any muscle, you need to keep using it for it to keep improving, so make sure that you work on maintaining and spreading positivity through the various aspects of your life.

Gratefulness is a fantastic way of turning negative thoughts into positive ones. You can even get a gratitude partner. Each of you creates lists in the mornings and/or evenings and then swaps them to experience one another's witnessing of possibilities and vision that surrounds you.

We can all overthink, but if you have a system to deal with it, you will be able to chase away the negativity that accompanies the habit of overthinking.

Chapter 6.

Common Questions and Misconceptions Surrounding NPD

In spite of the information provided in this book, there are still likely to be questions left unanswered. I know there are because I have taken a few choice questions that are asked often and may not have been fully, or directly, satisfied in the preluding discourse.

Narcissism has also gained a reputation as a Hollywood trope and now features predominantly in mass media as well as the younger generations' vocabulary. The word is tossed around as if it were a light weight to be applied liberally, and so misconceptions have naturally arrived. I will briefly touch on these before the conclusion.

This will be a small chapter dedicated to a handful of questions in the hopes of shedding more light on the subject.

How Do I Get Them to Change?

The short answer is that you don't, or you can't. Nobody is going to change just because you want them to, but instead, that need to change has to come from within themselves as it came from within you. The only changes in a person you truly can control are ones you make for yourself.

That being said, it is possible for narcissists to change but it is unlikely. Due to their nature, approaching a narcissist about their narcissism rarely bares fruit. If you and your significant other are able to broach the topic without the situation escalating then do so, otherwise, I strongly advise seeking out talk therapy through a certified professional.

They're Going to Call Again, What Do I Say or Do?

If you are already questioning the situation, I'd say you view it with apprehension, and you should block contact with that person immediately. The warning sign is you felt the need to ask this question because of what you were experiencing.

Maintaining no contact with the narcissist is the best way to handle any possible future encounter with them, especially if you never have to see them again. If, however, you have to deal with the narcissist regularly, keep the contact to a minimal. Remain polite but to the point on call, stick to the topic and don't get sucked into tangents, and always hold what is important to you to yourself, the narcissist doesn't need to know.

If There's Emotional or Psychological Abuse Involved, There Will Be Physical Abuse Too

This is not true. On the contrary, the reason that emotional and psychological abuse are so difficult to notice is because there are almost always no physical signs left behind. It takes a while for them to set in and they won't come in the shape of physical bruises, but rather in the form of bags under the victim's eyes, flinching at the sound of any raised voices, and the sudden withdrawal from things they used to enjoy, among other things. Knowing the signs is the only way to save yourself from or help someone else from the abusive cycle.

I Can't Deal with Silent Treatment and Stonewalling, Help

This is much like handling a narcissist when they petition you for contact through a message or a call; it's best to ignore it and get away from it if you can. Silent treatment is a powerful tool used as a form of manipulation by a narcissist with someone they know cares for them. They want you to get worked up and overreact and get tangled up tighter with them, but your best approach is to step back and away.

Silent treatment is a form of abuse and it is a tool, not a punishment that you earned or deserve. The narcissist is attempting to control you with this method and it's up to you to prevent that from happening.

Your best option is to get away. Stop contacting the person, stop seeing them, but rather move on with your life. If you show them how inconsequential their treatment is to your life, they will be the ones panicked and flustered.

If you are not able to leave or you share a common space such as a living area or work space, try and connect with someone else. This allows you to move on from the narcissist and thwart the effect they hoped the silent treatment would have on you.

Do Narcissists Adore Themselves?

The biggest misconception about narcissism is that every narcissist is a calloused individual who gains enjoyment from hurting others. While malignant narcissists may present as such, many narcissists were victims themselves. They have their own issues to deal with and their course of action is questionable, but it is not necessary to let their pain become your pain.

The reason the narcissist lashes out is because of how fragile they themselves are, and the pain they are experiencing can't be processed properly without them sharing suffering. A narcissist will appear on the surface as if they love nothing but themselves and spend half their day on their vanity alone, but under the surface there is a very different tale.

Most narcissists suffer from a heavy burden of insecurities, some of which tie in to the causality of their NPD. A narcissist is constantly comparing themselves to others and, if they don't measure up, they berate and belittle themselves. A narcissist damages more than just those around them.

Conclusion

U nless confronted, the pain of abuse can consume a victim. The hardest part about recovering from the cycle is to stop yourself from reflecting on what happened in the past and start focusing on the future instead; you don't have to settle for the past repeating itself just because you are afraid to be uncertain. Whether you are currently in the process of cutting off a narcissist or still making your way there, you are likely feeling a mix of confusing emotions—on the one hand, the narcissist may seem like an oppressor whilst on the other, you may find yourself glancing back wistfully at the person you thought they were.

Cognitive dissonance often goes hand-in-hand with abuse. It's the very thing that makes people not want to believe a victim who speaks out and it can cause the victim themselves to don rose-tinted glasses. An important step in overcoming this disbelief is to understand that narcissists don't change. Their personality disorder, as has been explained in this book, is something that they were born with. They are in the same category as other personality disorders such as sociopathy, histrionics, psychopaths, and borderline personality disorders.

This is literally who they are and who they have always been.

Your empathic nature is likely what led you to an abusive relationship. Not only do you attract the narcissist personality by nature, but your compassion and forgiveness repeatedly makes you give them the benefit of the doubt when they don't deserve it. Their behavior is thereby enabled and can even escalate from that point. That's not to say that your personality is a bad thing; only that it can be easily taken advantage of if you don't have the correct guards up. Now that you know more about them and how to catch the warning signs, you are better equipped. You can stop the abuse cycle from going full circle by replacing your unfailing kindness with firmer feet and an unwavering self-surety.

Turn all that care you had for someone who hurt you toward yourself. The first steps are always the hardest and you may find yourself stumbling and exhausted for a while, but each step you take adds up toward a journey. You've reached rock bottom and now it's time to climb out of there because the view from the top is good enough to keep you from ever spiraling down again. Your lifestyle should be one of self-devotion, self-care, and self-kindness. You can't fix other people, but you can fix yourself. Learn more about the person you are and make sure that you love them as hard as you can love others. Finding and putting yourself first are two of the best possible ways to break free from the codependent patterns that draw narcissists to you in the first place.

Once you start living, thinking, and feeling for yourself, you will find that abuse no longer finds you an appropriate target. Who knows? You might find yourself in a position like mine, where you can help others like yourself to transform and thrive after abuse. Don't leave it for next week. Start now and make self-care your default setting to see the true changes and feel the power of healing encompass you wholly.

If you felt this book helped you, reach out and let me know!

References

6 Ways to Stop Overthinking Everything. (2017). Inc.com. Retrieved from https://www.inc.com/amy-morin/6-ways-to-stop-overthinking-everything.html

10 Simple Ways You Can Stop Yourself From Overthinking. (2016). Inc.com. Retrieved from https://www.inc.com/lolly-daskal/10-simple-ways-you-can-stop-yourself-from-overthinking.html

7 benefits of having a hobby. (2019). positively present. Retrieved from https://www.positivelypresent.com/2013/06/benefits-of-having-a-hobby.html

Collingwood, J. (2016). Learning To Say No. Psych Central. Retrieved from https://psychcentral.com/lib/learning-to-say-no/

How and Why to Start Journaling. (2019). Lifehacker. Retrieved from https://lifehacker.com/why-you-should-keep-a-journal-and-how-to-start-yours-1547057185

4 Powerful Reasons to Meditate and How To Get Started | PickTheBrain | Motivation and Self Improvement. (2007). Pick the Brain | Motivation and Self Improvement. Retrieved from https://www.pickthebrain.com/blog/4-reasons-you-should-meditate-and-how-to-get-started/

Practicing Self-Care Is Important: 10 Easy Habits To Get You Started. (2019). Forbes.com. Retrieved from https://www.forbes.com/sites/payout/2017/09/19/practicing-self-care-is-important-10-easy-habits-to-get-you-started/#5efe081c283a

10 Steps to Getting Your Life Back After Narcissistic Abuse. (2018). Medium. Retrieved from https://medium.com/@SoulGPS/10-steps-to-getting-your-life-back-after-narcissistic-abuse-96b5c74af29c

4 Key Stages Of Healing After Narcissistic Abuse. (2018). Narcissism Recovery and Relationships Blog. Retrieved from https://blog.melanietoniaevans.com/4-key-stages-of-healing-after-narcissistic-abuse/

Gaslighting is the modern dating trend could leave you damaged. (2018). Mail Online. Retrieved from https://www.dailymail.co.uk/femail/article-5489585/Gaslighting-modern-dating-trend-leave-damaged.html

11 Warning Signs of Gaslighting. (2019). Psychology Today. Retrieved from https://www.psychologytoday.com/za/blog/here-there-and-everywhere/201701/11-warning-signs-gaslighting

How to Know If You're a Victim of Gaslighting. (2019). Psychology Today. Retrieved from https://www.psychologytoday.com/za/blog/toxic-relationships/201801/how-know-if-youre-victim-gaslighting

Luna, A. (2015). You're Not Going Crazy: 15 Signs You're a Victim of Gaslighting ★ LonerWolf. LonerWolf. Retrieved from https://lonerwolf.com/gaslighting/

Marie Hartwell-Walker, E. (2017). 7 Ways to Extinguish Gaslighting. World of Psychology. Retrieved from https://psychcentral.com/blog/7-ways-to-extinguish-gaslighting/

Gaslighting: 10 Signs You're Being Emotionally Abused | ThriveTalk. (2018). Thrivetalk. Retrieved from https://www.thrivetalk.com/gaslighting/

Help, G., Listed, G., Help, G., Therapist, F., Center, F., & Counselor, F. et al. (2018). Common Questions Asked by People Healing from Narcissistic Abuse. GoodTherapy.org Therapy Blog. Retrieved from https://www.goodtherapy.org/blog/common-questions-asked-by-people-healing-from-narcissistic-abuse-0507184

The Biggest Misconception about Narcissism - Kim Saeed: Narcissistic Abuse Recovery Program. (2017). Kim Saeed: Narcissistic Abuse Recovery Program. Retrieved from https://kimsaeed.com/2017/09/18/biggest-misconception-narcissism/

The Chaos Theory of Narcissistic Abuse - Kim Saeed: Narcissistic Abuse Recovery Program. (2017). Kim Saeed: Narcissistic Abuse Recovery Program. Retrieved from https://kimsaeed.com/2017/08/25/3-steps-freedom-times-emotional-chaos/

PTSD from Narcissistic Abuse - Kim Saeed: Narcissistic Abuse Recovery Program. (2014). Kim Saeed: Narcissistic Abuse Recovery Program. Retrieved from https://kimsaeed.com/2014/02/01/ptsd-in-the-aftermath-of-narcissistic-abuse/

Narcissistic personality disorder: Traits, diagnosis, and treatment. (2019). Medical News Today. Retrieved from https://www.medicalnewstoday.com/articles/9741.php#traits

6 Common Traits of Narcissists and Gaslighters. (2019). Psychology Today. Retrieved from https://www.psychologytoday.com/za/blog/communication-success/201707/6-common-traits-narcissists-and-gaslighters

9 Signs You're A Victim Of Narcissistic Abuse & Stuck In A Toxic Relationship. (2019). YourTango. Retrieved from https://www.yourtango.com/experts/joanne-brothwell/9-signs-toxic-relationship-suffering-narcissistic-abuse

Personality disorders - Symptoms and causes. (2019). Mayo Clinic. Retrieved from https://www.mayoclinic.org/diseases-conditions/personality-disorders/symptoms-causes/syc-20354463

Narcissistic personality disorder - Symptoms and causes. (2019). Mayo Clinic. Retrieved from https://www.mayoclinic.org/diseases-conditions/narcissistic-personality-disorder/symptoms-causes/syc-20366662

Narcissistic Personality Disorder. (2018). HelpGuide.org. Retrieved from https://www.helpguide.org/articles/mental-disorders/narcissistic-personality-disorder.htm

The Narcissistic Self (Everyday Narcissism) | Ridhwan. (2019). Diamondapproach.org. Retrieved from https://www.diamondapproach.org/blog/narcissistic-self-everyday-narcissism?utm_source=google&utm_medium=ad%20grant&utm_campaign=narcissism&gclid=Cj0KCQjwrrXtBRCKARIs

AMbU6bHWydxjJ93qoD2Mk6A65ccntfviDhpFhOAPnde6bk
1-l874PDAqLIgaAiNGEALw_wcB

Our Three Brains - The Reptilian Brain. (2017). The
Interaction Design Foundation. Retrieved from
https://www.interaction-design.org/literature/article/our-three-brains-the-reptilian-brain

Hypomania and mania | Mind, the mental health charity - help
for mental health problems. (2019). Mind.org.uk. Retrieved
from https://www.mind.org.uk/information-support/types-of-mental-health-problems/hypomania-and-mania/#.XdJJod7zmUn

Narcissistic personality disorder: Traits, diagnosis, and
treatment. (2019). Medical News Today. Retrieved from
https://www.medicalnewstoday.com/articles/9741.php

Narcissistic Personality Disorder: Practice Essentials,
Background, Pathophysiology and Etiology. (2019).
Emedicine.medscape.com. Retrieved from
https://emedicine.medscape.com/article/1519417-overview#a1

Kristen Milstead, P., & Kristen Milstead, P. (2018). 8 Types of
Narcissists- Including One to Stay Away From at All Costs.
Mindcology. Retrieved from
https://mindcology.com/narcissist/8-types-narcissists-including-one-stay-away-costs/

Luna, A. (2016). Dear Empaths: 4 Types of Narcissists You
May Be Attracting ★ LonerWolf. LonerWolf. Retrieved from
https://lonerwolf.com/empaths-and-narcissists/

Avoid all 6 types of narcissists—but mental-health pros say one type is especially damaging. (2019). Well+Good. Retrieved from https://www.wellandgood.com/good-advice/types-of-narcissists/

5 Types of Extreme Narcissists (and How to Deal With Them). (2019). Psychology Today. Retrieved from https://www.psychologytoday.com/us/blog/shame/201509/5-types-extreme-narcissists-and-how-deal-them

4 Types of Narcissist, and How to Spot Each One. (2019). Psychology Today. Retrieved from https://www.psychologytoday.com/za/blog/i-hear-you/201904/4-types-narcissist-and-how-spot-each-one

11 Signs You're The Victim of Narcissistic Abuse. (2017). Thought Catalog. Retrieved from https://thoughtcatalog.com/shahida-arabi/2017/11/11-devastating-signs-youve-been-abused-by-a-malignant-narcissist/

The little-known reasons why you need to leave the narcissist ASAP! - Kim Saeed: Narcissistic Abuse Recovery Program. (2016). Kim Saeed: Narcissistic Abuse Recovery Program. Retrieved from https://kimsaeed.com/2016/01/17/the-little-known-reasons-why-you-need-to-leave-the-narcissist-asap/

11 Signs You're Dating a Narcissist — and How to Deal with Them. (2019). Healthline. Retrieved from https://www.healthline.com/health/mental-health/am-i-dating-a-narcissist#1

How to Overcome Fear After Psychological Narcissistic Abuse - Kim Saeed: Narcissistic Abuse Recovery Program. (2019).

Kim Saeed: Narcissistic Abuse Recovery Program. Retrieved from https://kimsaeed.com/2019/01/22/how-to-overcome-fear-after-psychological-narcissistic-abuse/

The Wounded Child: 7 Needs Narcissistic Parents Cannot Provide - Kim Saeed: Narcissistic Abuse Recovery Program. (2018). Kim Saeed: Narcissistic Abuse Recovery Program. Retrieved from https://kimsaeed.com/2018/10/09/the-wounded-child-7-needs-narcissistic-parents-cannot-provide/

Working The 5 Phases of Trauma Recovery After Narcissistic Abuse - Kim Saeed: Narcissistic Abuse Recovery Program. (2018). Kim Saeed: Narcissistic Abuse Recovery Program. Retrieved from https://kimsaeed.com/2018/08/01/working-the-5-phases-of-trauma-recovery-after-narcissistic-abuse/

HuffPost is now a part of Verizon Media. (2019). Huffpost.com. Retrieved from https://www.huffpost.com/entry/signs-of-narcissism_n_5a26cf6de4b069df71fa196b

Hypomania and mania | Mind, the mental health charity - help for mental health problems. (2019). Mind.org.uk. Retrieved from https://www.mind.org.uk/information-support/types-of-mental-health-problems/hypomania-and-mania/#.XdJLi97zmUl

The Cognitive Neuroscience of Narcissism. (2018). Journal Of Brain, Behaviour And Cognitive Sciences, 1(1). Retrieved from http://www.imedpub.com/articles/the-cognitive-neuroscience-of-narcissism.php?aid=22149

Darlene Lancer, M. (2016). What is Narcissistic Abuse?.
Psych Central. Retrieved from
https://psychcentral.com/lib/what-is-narcissistic-abuse/

J, R. (2019). Narcissism and the use of fantasy. - PubMed -
NCBI . Ncbi.nlm.nih.gov. Retrieved from
https://www.ncbi.nlm.nih.gov/pubmed/1939692

How the Stories We Tell Ourselves Build or Relieve Anxiety
— My Wellbeing. (2018). My Wellbeing. Retrieved from
https://mywellbeing.com/therapy-101/2018/8/22/how-the-
stories-we-tell-ourselves-build-or-relieve-anxiety

Understanding the Mind of a Narcissist . (2019). Psychology
Today. Retrieved from
https://www.psychologytoday.com/intl/blog/toxic-
relationships/201804/understanding-the-mind-narcissist

The Narcissist's Grandiose Fantasies | HealthyPlace. (2019).
Healthyplace.com. Retrieved from
https://www.healthyplace.com/personality-
disorders/malignant-self-love/narcissists-grandiose-fantasies

10 Ways To Stand Your Ground When You're STUCK With A
Narcissist. (2016). YourTango. Retrieved from
https://www.yourtango.com/experts/elizabethstone/how-cope-
narcissist-who-youre-stuck

How to Deal with Emotional Abuse | Crisis Text Line . (2019).
Crisis Text Line. Retrieved 18 November 2019, from
https://www.crisistextline.org/get-help/emotional-abuse